Healthy Living

Prolonging Life Span

I0415528

Introduction

I want to thank you and congratulate you for downloading the book, *"Healthy living"*.

This book contains proven steps and strategies on how to lead an healthy living.

Healthy living is following some rules in order to make our life simple and long. These rules are no rocket science and every one can follow provided one does with dedication. Great people don't do great things to become great. But they do things differently. The key to find the treasure of healthy living is being moderate. Paying attention to economic aspect, diet, exercise, sleep and shelter can lead to a prolonged lifespan. It is indeed a golden era where there are no dearth of medical resources. At every step when there is an alarm on the health issue, we are able to deal it with the immediate medical aid available. Still as the saying goes, 'Prevention is better than cure'. Therefore, for a healthy living and a prolonging lifespan, some simple yet significant measures can be taken. We can make our lives fit and healthy.

Thanks again for downloading this book, I hope you enjoy its style

information is without contract or any type of guarantee assurance.

The trademarks that are used are without any consent, and the publication of the trademark is without permission or backing by the trademark owner. All trademarks and brands within this book are for clarifying purposes only and are the owned by the owners themselves, not affiliated with this document.

Chapter 1
Healthy living
Prolonging lifespan

Healthy living is a lifestyle. It is an orderly living for the longevity of life. We find many people living beyond 80 years. When we happen to peep into their lives, a common thing which is leading to longevity is moderation. When we notice the factors which can be acclimatized in life, some of the crucial factors included in the prolonged lifespan are:

a. Economic aspects
b. Diet
c. Exercise
d. Sleep
e. Shelter

Moderation in the above mentioned areas can lead to a win-win situation of life. An ideal way of nurturing the treasure of life is to lead in a simple manner yet be moderate. The secrets of life are explored in the simplicity adhered in living. This can be viewed as the most diligent and unbelievable task of healthy living. But, in fact it can be generalized knowing the lives of people who have lived a long life.

Economic aspects play an important role in our life. Investment in education is said to be the best form of investment. Education shape up our lives to a better human being. We earn to handle necessities of our life and our family. Our budget caters to the diet we have, house we live. Wise allocation of money into the priorities of life will reap the benefits.

Diet is the most important aspect of life. Balanced diet sustain a prolonged life. Nutrition and health play hand in hand. Good Nutrition is good health. Awareness of good diet is the need of an hour. People walk in to trouble when they face the adversities of wrong diet, i.e. junk food, too
spicy food, alcohol etc.

Exercise adds glow to life. They aid in smooth functioning of our physical and mental health. Exercise make us fit and healthy enough to capture the essence of life with ease. It is an important parameter of quality of life. There are many breathing techniques which can make our lives stress free. In addition, there are number of therapeutic uses of few exercises. Exercises provide pillars of strength, flexibility and endurance to the body. It eliminates excess body fat and gives form to the body. It helps in prolonging life. It can contribute for a healthy weight, maintaining healthy bone density, muscle strength, mobility of joints, strengthening the immune system. Exercise increases the life expectancy and prevents aging.

Sleep is the crucial factor for leading a good life. 6-8 hours of sleep is the essential requirement for a fresh day. During sleep the brain sorts and processes the information. It is essential to create long term memories as the brain takes up all information of the day and stores, to be used later. Inadequate sleep will trigger irritation and disturbance for a person when he is set out for work.

Shelter is the basic human requirement. Living in a aerated house will stimulate good health. It will cater to good sleep. A proper shelter accommodates fresh air and help in preserving the physical and mental health.

These factors will keep the energy level at high pace and keep our stamina to fit the profession and come out with flying colors. It has been found that when diet, exercise and sleep of children were taken into consideration. They were able to grasp the learn better. It gave a remarkable affect on their performance. Children have found to score better a in their academic pursuits and sports too. Teachers who paid attention to their diet, exercise and sleep were found to teach better. In fact, good teaching learning atmosphere was developed in the curriculum. Not only in the teaching profession people in different professions found improved performance in their respective fields who catered to the dimensions of healthy diet, exercise and good sleep As the people prone to pay attention to the above set of guidelines they were found to be passionate about their professional life as well as personal life.

Many people have found to excel in their life by laying the foundation of some of the principles. Food is body, body is mind, mind is food. Food is found to affect in the body. Fresh food leads to healthy body and healthy body leads to a healthy mind. A healthy mind influences vibrates the food. Just as we find the food in temple or a holy place carrying divinity. Similarly, a healthy mind influences the food. It is a vicious circle.

Care, love and attention to the elderly can help them to have interest in the life. It is found young people can take care of themselves. Children are taken care by parents. But parents find difficulty to take care of elders. Being affectionate to the feeling of the elderly and senior citizens can create zeal in their lives. The timely medication, care can help to sustain their lives. Life is a bundle of joy and experiences of one another creating a cluster affect of share and care among individuals. It is this share and care which is considered as very precious and valuable.

Now-a-days people from children to elders are affected by online games. Games are a source of recreation when play moderately. Elders are also finding some games very interesting like Candy crush, Township, Clash of cans, Pubg game etc. But when played extremely it is causing anxiety, anger and several other symptoms. There are several other source of entertainment which people find themselves to be in par. These include YouTube channels, where people watch videos related to their interest. There are tons of channels of health and they follow the information and are guided to good health.

Another area of concern is the mental health of an Individual. In school, colleges and offices, we find people diving into the depths of depression. A sadness which persists for a very long time. When such situation arises then the person in not healthy though he may look physically healthy. Such people have suicidal tendencies. Proper counseling and medication can help the person to come out of depression.

According World Health Organization who has defined health as, 'a state of complete physical, mental and social well-being and not merely the absence of disease or infirmity'. The factors of healthy living mentioned in this chapter play simple yet significant role in healthy living.

Society can help person to lead a normal life by accepting the person. Emotional support and having empathy to the person helps the person recover from mental illness. Besides medication also proves for improvement in the mental health. There are many celebrities who have been suffering from depression. Some of them are Selena Gomez, Jim Carrey, Beyoncé, Deepika Padukone, Carrie Fisher have spoken about their issues of depression, anxiety and mental health. Family support and medication have helped them to come out of their illness.

Healthy living is related to physical, mental and social health. When a person in healthy in these domains, there can be a prolonging lifespan

Points to remember
- **Healthy living**
- **Economic aspects, diet, exercise, sleep and shelter are the important factors for a healthy living.**

Chapter 2
Economic aspects

How can economic aspects lead to a healthy living? This question's lies in the fact that to lead a life, economic factors play an crucial role.

We need not become Mark Zuckerberg or Mukesh Ambani to stay healthy. We can be healthy with the domains of finance within our own range. Unlimited talk time is given by few companies but can we guarantee unlimited health of our lives. We can guarantee and take charge to optimize the parameters of health for a prolonged life. What ever lifespan we have it is upon us to extend the validity through our willpower. It is a magnificent power almighty has given to uplift ourselves and uplift the people around who so ever require help. Through the finance what we have, we can plan and prepare for a life of longevity.

People spend lots of money to lead a happy life, but they need not land healthily. In fact, money can lead to an obese and diseased life too. Many people are often found to break the rules and land up in crimes. Money can lead to egoist tendency in people. Money can lead people to lose importance on the value of small things. It can lead in taking things for granted. Money can lead to people to absorb the values like corruption and malpractices. There are people who spend lavishing and end up in depts. It has been found that urban people having good jobs are flooded with loans which is leading to urban poverty. History showed people who were once into name and fame but still have landed into misfortune by their lavish lifestyles. Michael Jackson, a famous singer who had many million fans also had the money factor not properly handed and had been into debts. A famous South Indian celebrity and film star of the seventy's, Mrs. Savithri also went through numerous trouble as she was not able to manage and invest it properly. Lives of many more people are an example to learn how careful it is to manage money. Money is a substance which requires spending very systematically, weighing the pros and cons. Therefore, people should maintain economic balance systematically. Money is not everything but a tool to get something in life. So, wise spending when required can lead a happy and prosperous home.

A happy home requires money for their monthly expenses, medical expenses, home rents, petrol expenses and recreation. Balanced and calculated expenses in relation to their budget can lead for a joyful and happy home. Hence, it is absolutely necessary for a moderation in economic aspects. Money has invisible legs to run so it doesn't stays at one place. It firmly stays, if earned with noble deeds. Hard work and smart work give money. Wise spending of money can help in safe and secure life. Qualitative spending of money can lead to a life of harmony and a prolonged lifespan.

People are bound to worship money as it opens the doors of prosperity. But now-a-days, it is settling in the minds of people. People are ingrained with the idea that money can buy everything. A false notion that is instilled on them. But, the fact is it is guide for a healthy life.

Wise guidelines of the family budget allocation to proper diet, good house and other necessary requirement can help in a healthy lifestyle. It is seen that rejuvenation of the thoughts arise when the mind is still and calm. Therefore, exercise and relaxation techniques done this moment invest the profits of whole day with active energy.

Periodic checking and examination of the parameters like blood sugar, urine, cholesterol also are the indicators of healthy living. As prevention is better than cure. Therefore, monitoring the health is also an added dimension of being cautiously healthy.

Few people also get operated when they happen to know that they might get a particular disease which has been hereditary one. Angelina Jolie also had undergone operation and got her ovary removed, as she knew about the history of ovarian cancer in her family.

Healthy living defines the role played by people in leading a happy living with good health, physical, mental and social. By good health their lifespan is prolonging. The economic aspects do influence our health. As the health checkup do costs money and to meet the medical expenses we require adequate finance. Therefore adequate planning of financial resources are required to branch the various priorities, necessary expenses like medical treatment etc.

Points to remember

1. It is right thinking mind-→money--→ diet, exercise, sleep, shelter → healthy life.
2. Periodic health checkup will sustain good health

Chapter 3

Diet

Balanced Diet is the term often heard and seen. It is a resource entering the body to energize and to keep healthy. Nutritious food keep the spirit high. But, if the food is not taken moderately can lead to cause diseases. If people crave for junk food they naturally become obese. Besides, eating sugary foods like ice-creams, sweets can make people diabetic. Sometimes, other reasons of getting diabetes, have also been found. Food can be a source of disappointment as people crave and are unable to remain fit. In fact, weight management is the talk of town. Either overweight or underweight and they are unable to maintain their ideal weight. The exercise and slimming centre's are mushrooming today because people are having food but unable to control their weight. Apps related to health, exercise are installed by people in their phones to cater the health issues. If food is taken scarcely, people suffer from malnutrition and becoming anemic.

Vegetarian or non-vegetarian is another question?

People often raise their eyebrow on which diet to follow. Whichever diet we follow moderation is of utmost importance.

Drink or not?

Another popular question. If people cannot avoid alcohol, they can drink moderately. Not deviating from binge drinking once in a month or in weekends. If people are not used to drinking, it is well and good.

A good diet should contain carbohydrates, proteins and fats. Apart from this minerals and vitamins are also equally important. Some of the sources of good diet are green leafy vegetables, eggs, fish, cereals, sprouts, milk, honey, fruits etc. A diet also has the potentiality to drive away harmful disease causing germs like bacteria and viruses. It also creates resistance in the body and prevents diseases.

For the weight loss issues various diets have come up in the recent times. Some of them are:

1. Ketogenic diet
2. OMAD diet(One Meal a Day)
3. Paleo diet
4. Vegetarian diet
5. Vegan diet
6. Raw food diet

People have adopted these diets and have found to useful for weight loss.

A diet is also classified according to yoga in terms of

1. Satvik diet
2. Rajasic diet
3. Tamasic diet

1. Satvik diet: It tends to keep the mind active and calm. It helps to do the daily practice of Meditation. It includes fresh food cooked from vegetables, rice.

2. Rajasic diet: It creates turbulence in mind. It gives more energy to the body and mind. Such diet helps to adapt to the lifestyle having more of physical and mental activity. It includes garlic, onions, spicy food.

3. Tamasic diet: It creates dullness in mind. It gives energy but the tendency of sleep is associated with the food after we eat. It includes non-vegetarian food, curd, fermented food.

It is upon us to decide which diet to pickup according to our lifestyle. In earlier days and even today, people who lead a life with meditation as a practice follow satvik diet. It helps to lead a life where some of the values like forgiveness, compassion, peace, goodness are instilled.

People who are involved in profession like army, police where protecting the people of the nation is their priority they are focused to shoot the enemy or the terrorists. Such people have the dare and stare the enemy to keep them at bay. Rajasic diet is good for such people where physical and mental activity are at an extreme end. There is tendency of eye for an eye attitude among individuals.

Tamasic diet is good for people who consume food to get energy. People feel the energy but after a period of lag or nap. It is creates lethargy. The attitude towards life is negative.

The types of foods also leads to different types of behaviors among people. Satvik food favor pious behavior, rajasic food favor fighting tendencies and tamasic food favor not willing behavior. As the saying in Bible goes, Food becomes flesh. Therefore the food we have manifests in the body and behavior of the person. We can set the guidelines of the type of behavior which we aspire and have that type of food.

Points to remember

- Balanced diet should contain carbohydrates, proteins, fats, minerals and vitamins.
- Diet is also classified into satvik, rajasic and tamasic.

Chapter 4

Exercise

Exercise creates the healthy body. Exercise maintains physical fitness. It helps to radiate an active personality. Exercise helps in productions of endorphins in the neuro-secretory cells. People feel more happier when they make exercise a part and parcel of their lifestyle. It stimulates the metabolism. It makes the body fit and healthy. It strengthens and tones muscles. It enhances pumping of bloods to every part of body. It floods the oxygen supply to each and every tissue of our body. People have been found to look ageless through exercise.

There are people who run, walk to keep themselves healthy. Besides some others swim. Some of them find sports the best form of physical activity to stay healthy. Some others do martial arts to remain fit. Some prefer weight training. Some do yoga to increase their flexibility. Some of the exercises are also have the capacity to cure diseases of people. Besides different exercises can be done to cure specific disease.

Aerobic exercises include running, cycling, brisk walking, continuous training etc. It increases cardiovascular endurance. Anaerobic exercises include weight training, interval training, functional training etc. It tones muscles and improves bone strength. Flexibility exercises stretch and length muscles. It improves joint flexibility and keep muscles fit.

Martial Arts are practiced for physical and mental alertness. It is a form of self-defense. I was called as the combat systems. It is the art of fighting. Through the practice of Martial arts there is a boost in the strength, stamina, speed, flexibility, movement and coordination.

Number of areas where people plunge to rescue are growing day by day are solace to peace. In this regard, many people find relaxation techniques and meditation and Yoga extremely helpful. It is silencing the mind to get prepared to new challenges ahead. These have also found to be a major factor in the prolonging lifespan. It is yoga which helps to the union of body with the Almighty. The various poses of yoga have been found to be extremely beneficial. Besides physical benefits, it also calms the mind. It is also aids in weight loss and flexibility. Some of the breathing techniques like Pranayama, Bhastrika Bhramri Pranayama have been found useful to calm the mind.

Whichever is the form of exercise the motto is good health. It is of immense joy that through few poses we can achieve energy and long lasting health. It is powerful as it carries the fragment of life towards longevity.

Points to remember

1. Exercise is a key to sustain good health
2. It helps in flexibility and to remain fit.

Chapter 5

Sleep

Good Sleep leads to good health. People know this fact but still tend to shudder the importance of sleep. Sleep is a crucial aspect of a healthy life. Too much sleep tend to make a fresh morning lethargic and dull. Less sleep tend to make a tiresome and irritating morning. 6-8 hours of sound sleep is an ideal one for good health.

Another question is to get up early or not?

There are tons of arguments in this regard. Some people are in favor of early rise while some people strongly believe to get up late. Whichever is the case one can make sure that 6-8 hours of sound sleep is there. One cannot deny that health benefits of people who early morning are more while compared to people who get up late. However, it is up to people to choose to get up early or late depending on their lifestyle but most crucial is moderation in sleep and

6-8 hours of sound sleep. If less sleep with sound and good sleep is there, it will also fetch active morning.

People now-a-days are adopting nocturnal style of living. They are more active in the midnight and do their work amidst the nocturnal arena. Such people wake up by 10 a.m. and do their morning tasks. While there are many jobs having night shifts and people work at night and sleep in the day. In fact, in some places people go out to eat in the broad midnight. There are crowds of people too having food at midnight in the streets. Specific food stalls in Vijayawada, Andhra Pradesh display the food items at night. People flourish at night to enjoy food. Its changing time and picking up our choice of sleeping time according to our schedule.

REM(rapid eye movement) and non-REM are the two phases of sleep. During sleep the body systems are in an anabolic state. Sleep restores the different immune systems, nervous, skeletal and muscular systems in the body. The circadian clock provides sleep at night. It is found that the brain utilizes less energy while sleeping than when awake. Sleep facilitates the synthesis of molecules to repair and protect brain from harmful elements generated during awake state of brain. There are people suffering from insomnia or sleeping disorders. Deprivation of sleep may impair the body's ability to heal wounds. It also impairs the immune function. There are medication available for the treatment of these disorders. Sleep difficulties are associated with disorders such as depression, bi-polar disorder etc. It has been found that sleeping 6-7 hours each night will lead to prolonged lifespan and good cardiac health. Sleep varies with age and among individuals.

People can choose the lifestyle comfortable for them but only thing they can ensure is that to have a sound sleep.

Points to remember

1. 6-8 hours of sound sleep is vital for life

Chapter 6

Shelter

Shelter refers to the basic need of life to protect from animals, heat, cold weather and rain. It is one of the component to stay healthy. A home is a place where we live. A home is to cherish the moments of life. A house well ventilated will make the people diseased free. A house having the necessary facilities will help to have good sleep and a healthy atmosphere. A house located near a polluted area can make ill health. Likewise, houses placed where there is too much noise will make people prone to different health issues.

Many disease like mumps, chicken pox, malaria, dengue fever spread rapidly because of unhygienic conditions pertaining to the household. Some of them become epidemic and affect large number of people. Several bacterial diseases like cholera, diphtheria, whooping cough, leprosy, spread due to contamination of air, water and food. Some of the viral diseases prominent are common cold, chicken pox, mumps, AIDS, hepatitis.

Ascariasis, Schistosomiasis, taeniasis are some infections caused by worms. Mosquitoes cause diseases like malaria, filaria etc. Amoebiasis or amoebic dysentery is another disease caused by single celled entamoeba. Proper vaccination measure to children can help to control the disease. Hence the home we stay, safe water to drink are of prior requirement. Care has to be taken regarding the surrounding. Neat and clean home and its surrounding is also an indicator of good health. Well maintained house with greenery are the reflection of a healthy person. Plants are source of oxygen and more greenery enhances the oxygen in the air. Planting trees and developing green belt in our surrounding foster good health. It attracts more of biodiversity. Birds and butterflies move around. Many people are planting sapling on their birthdays. This culture is indeed very welcoming. One can increase the greenery through the plantation in their surrounding. When people are responsible for the growing plants, everyone is benefited by the oxygen.

People live in different types of houses according to their needs, i.e. Wooden house, brick house, glass house etc. Some live in independent house, some in apartments, some others in huts. Few people have their vanity van designed as a house to meet their needs. Few others have houses in boats. Few others have planes designed as home and office for their convenience. Which ever is the case the basic amenities of good health and hygiene are to taken care of.

Points to remember
1. Place to reside which is well ventilated.
2. Good house will keep good health.

Conclusion

Health is a boon in our hands. A cautious attention to the diet, exercise, sleep and shelter can help in the prolonging lifespan. Having every thing in life will not lead to success, as a heap of stones will not make a house. A systematic construction of house with bricks and cement will make a house. Similarly, a systematic planning in the factors like economy, diet, exercise, sleep and shelter will lead in a prolonging lifespan. The economic areas are to be planned and diet, exercise, adequate sleep and shelter are catered to have a significance in healthy living. Proper dietary measures can sustain with healthy body and fitness can be achieved by exercise. With good and sound sleep one can feel fresh with full energy. Prolonging lifespan are a matter of sustaining the energy our treasure to its optimum. Everyone can achieve it provided they follow the important factors mentioned in this book.

Thank you again for downloading this book!

I hope this book was able to help you to know the ways of healthy living. In this book one can find all the possibilities of prolonging life span.

The next step is to cater to the moderation in life. Life is filled with possibilities and the moderation in the aspects mentioned in the book one can pave the rods to healthy living.

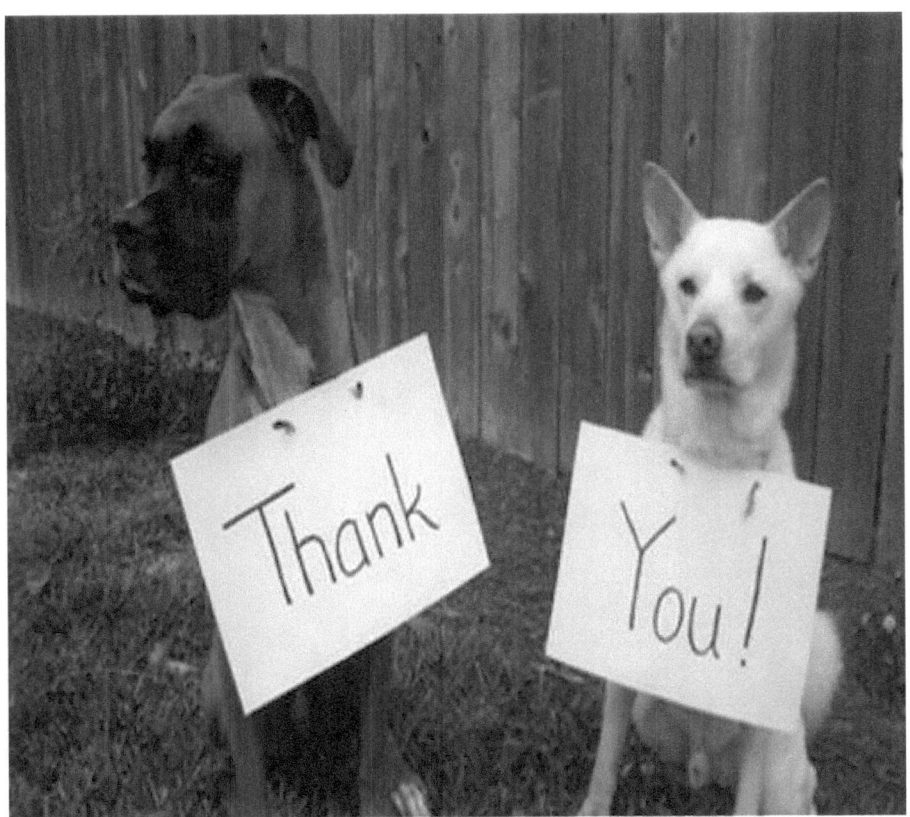

Finally, if you enjoyed this book, then I'd like to ask you for a favor, would you be kind enough to leave a review for this book on Amazon? It'd be greatly appreciated!

Thank you and good luck!